UNDERSTANDING
PROBIOTICS
AND BENEFITS

A Guide To Boost Your Immunity, Grasp The Major Targets, Focus, And Key Points For Optimal Health

DR. LACEY MICHELLE

Disclaimer:

The information provided in this book is for general informational purposes only and is not intended as medical advice.

Readers are encouraged to consult with a qualified healthcare professional for any health concerns or questions.

The author of this book is not affiliated with any individual, website, organization, or products mentioned within.

This book does not endorse or promote any specific brands, services, or external entities. Any references made are purely for illustrative purposes and should not be construed as endorsements.

Readers are responsible for their own decisions and should conduct their own research before making any health-related choices.

Any liability resulting from the use of this information, whether direct or indirect, is disclaimed by the author and publisher.

Contents

About This Book:

Probiotics as a Supplement: Nourishing Your Gut for Optimal Health" delves into the world of probiotics, offering a comprehensive exploration of their definition, types, and historical significance. This book aims to unravel the science behind probiotics, shedding light on their role in microorganisms, mechanisms of action, and the distinction between probiotics and prebiotics.

Understanding Probiotics

Definition and Types

Historical Perspective

Importance in Gut Health

The Science Behind Probiotics

CHAPTER ONE

What Are Probiotics?

Probiotics, a term often heard in the context of health and wellness, refer to live microorganisms that offer a range of potential health benefits when consumed in adequate amounts.

These microorganisms are typically bacteria or yeasts that can help maintain or restore a balanced microbial environment in the gut, known as the gut microbiome. The term "probiotic" is derived from the Greek words "pro" and "biotic," which mean "for life." Essentially, probiotics are living organisms that are beneficial for human life and well-being.

Defining Probiotics

Probiotics are often defined as "good" or "friendly" bacteria that promote a harmonious coexistence with the trillions of microorganisms that inhabit the human gastrointestinal tract.

These microorganisms aid in various essential functions, such as digestion, nutrient absorption, immune system modulation, and protection against harmful pathogens. Probiotics work by competitively excluding harmful microbes, stimulating the production of beneficial molecules, and enhancing the gut's barrier function. They are considered a vital component of the gut-brain axis, influencing both physical and mental health.

Probiotic products are widely available in various forms, including supplements, fermented foods, and certain dairy products like yogurt. The two most common probiotic genera are Lactobacillus and Bifidobacterium, though other strains like Saccharomyces boulardii are also recognized for their potential health benefits. Probiotic supplements, in particular, have gained popularity as a convenient way to introduce specific strains of beneficial microorganisms into the gut.

History Of Probiotic Use

The concept of using live microorganisms to promote health dates back to ancient civilizations. Fermented foods, which contain naturally occurring probiotics, have been part of human diets for thousands of years. Historical records indicate that cultures like the Greeks and Romans, as well as Asian civilizations, were well aware of the benefits of fermented foods for digestive health.

The modern understanding of probiotics can be traced to the early 20th century, with the work of Elie Metchnikoff, a Nobel Prize-winning scientist. Metchnikoff proposed the idea that the consumption of fermented dairy products, such as yogurt, contributed to the longevity of Bulgarian peasants. This observation sparked further scientific interest in probiotics and their potential to influence health. Over time, research has led to a better understanding of the specific strains and mechanisms behind probiotic benefits.

Types Of Probiotic Strains

Probiotics encompass a diverse range of bacterial and yeast strains, each with its unique properties and potential health effects. Two of the most well-known genera of probiotics are Lactobacillus and Bifidobacterium. These genera consist of multiple species and strains, such as Lactobacillus acidophilus, Lactobacillus rhamnosus, and Bifidobacterium bifidum, to name a few. Each strain may offer distinct advantages, with some being more effective in treating specific conditions or supporting various aspects of health.

In addition to Lactobacillus and Bifidobacterium, other probiotic strains like Saccharomyces boulardii, a yeast, have gained recognition for their ability to prevent and manage gastrointestinal issues, including diarrhea and irritable bowel syndrome. Furthermore, there are probiotic combinations formulated to provide a wider spectrum of benefits by incorporating multiple strains with complementary actions.

Understanding the diversity of probiotic strains and their specific applications is essential for tailoring probiotic supplementation to individual health needs.

Different strains may be more effective in addressing conditions like irritable bowel syndrome, allergies, or even enhancing immune system function.

Consequently, the selection of a probiotic supplement should be based on a clear understanding of the desired health outcomes and the scientific evidence supporting the chosen strains.

probiotics are live microorganisms that play a crucial role in maintaining a balanced gut microbiome and promoting overall health. With a history dating back thousands of years, the use of probiotics has evolved from traditional fermented foods to modern probiotic supplements.

The diversity of probiotic strains, such as Lactobacillus, Bifidobacterium, and

Saccharomyces boulardii, offers a wide range of potential health benefits. As research in this field continues to expand, the understanding of probiotics and their applications in healthcare will likely continue to evolve, offering new possibilities for improving human well-being.

How Probiotics Work

Probiotics are living microorganisms that can provide numerous health benefits when consumed in adequate amounts. They primarily consist of beneficial bacteria and some yeasts that naturally inhabit our gastrointestinal tract.

These microorganisms play a crucial role in maintaining the delicate balance of our gut microbiome and have far-reaching effects on various aspects of our health.

Gut-Brain Connection

The gut-brain connection is a fascinating and intricate concept that highlights the bidirectional communication between our gut and brain. Probiotics are known to influence this connection in several ways.

The gut is often referred to as the "second brain" because it contains an extensive network of neurons, and it produces neurotransmitters that impact our mood and behavior. Probiotics can positively affect this gut-brain axis by modulating the gut microbiota composition and thus influencing neurotransmitter production. This has led to research into the potential of probiotics in improving mood, reducing stress, and even managing certain mental health conditions.

Probiotics play a crucial role in supporting our immune system. A significant portion of our immune system resides in the gut, where it interacts with the vast and diverse community of microorganisms.

Probiotics can enhance our immune defenses by promoting the growth of beneficial bacteria, which can compete with harmful pathogens for resources and produce compounds that stimulate the immune system.

They also help maintain the integrity of the intestinal barrier, preventing harmful substances from leaking into the bloodstream, which could trigger immune responses.

Probiotics are often used to support immune function, especially during times of illness or following antibiotic treatment, which can disrupt the gut microbiome.

Fermentation And Digestion

Fermentation is a key process in the breakdown of complex carbohydrates in the gut, and probiotics are actively involved in this process.

These beneficial microorganisms can ferment certain dietary fibers, resulting in the production of short-chain fatty acids (SCFAs), such as butyrate, acetate, and propionate. SCFAs serve as an energy source for the cells lining the colon and contribute to gut health.

Additionally, probiotics aid in the digestion and absorption of nutrients, particularly lactose and certain vitamins. Individuals with lactose intolerance or specific nutrient absorption issues may benefit from the use of probiotics to alleviate digestive discomfort.

Preventing Pathogenic Overgrowth

Pathogenic microorganisms, often referred to as "bad bacteria," can pose a threat to our health when they overgrow in the gut. Probiotics act as a natural defense mechanism against pathogenic overgrowth by competing for space and resources within the gut environment.

They help maintain a balanced microbial community, preventing the harmful bacteria from gaining a foothold. Probiotics also produce antimicrobial compounds that inhibit the growth of pathogenic bacteria.

This protective role is particularly important in preventing conditions such as bacterial overgrowth syndrome, which can lead to digestive problems and other health issues.

probiotics are a valuable tool in promoting overall health by influencing the gut-brain connection, supporting the immune system, aiding in fermentation and digestion, and preventing pathogenic overgrowth.

Their role in maintaining a harmonious gut microbiome underscores their importance in various aspects of health, and ongoing research continues to uncover the full extent of their potential benefits.

CHAPTER TWO

The Benefits Of Probiotics

Probiotics, living microorganisms that provide health benefits when consumed in adequate amounts, have gained increasing attention and popularity due to their potential positive impact on various aspects of human health. These microscopic organisms, primarily bacteria and some yeasts, offer a wide array of advantages, including improvements in digestive health, immune system support, mental well-being, skin health, women's health, and even the management of allergies and asthma.

Digestive Health

One of the most well-known benefits of probiotics is their role in promoting digestive health. Probiotics help maintain a balanced gut microbiome by increasing the population of beneficial bacteria and suppressing the growth of harmful microorganisms. This balance in the gut can alleviate common digestive issues, such as bloating, gas, diarrhea, and constipation.

Probiotics are often recommended to individuals suffering from conditions like irritable bowel syndrome (IBS) and inflammatory bowel diseases (IBD) like Crohn's disease and ulcerative colitis.

Immune System Support

The gut plays a vital role in the body's immune system, and a balanced gut microbiome is essential for optimal immune function. Probiotics can enhance the body's immune response by promoting the production of antibodies and other immune cells. Regular consumption of probiotics may reduce the risk of infections and improve the body's ability to fight off pathogens. It's important to note that different strains of probiotics can have varying effects on the immune system, making it essential to choose the right strains for specific health goals.

Probiotics And Mental Health

The gut-brain connection is a fascinating area of research, and it is increasingly recognized that the gut microbiome can influence mental health. Probiotics have shown promise in potentially alleviating symptoms of mood disorders, anxiety, and depression. The gut microbiome communicates with the brain through the gut-brain axis, and probiotics may help regulate this connection. While more research is needed to fully understand the mechanisms at play, the potential link between probiotics and mental well-being is an exciting area of study.

Skin Health

Probiotics may not only have internal health benefits but also play a role in maintaining healthy skin. Skin conditions like acne, eczema, and rosacea are often associated with imbalances in the gut microbiome. Probiotics can help modulate the immune response and inflammation, which can contribute to the management of these skin conditions.

Some skincare products even incorporate probiotics to promote a balanced skin microbiome and improve overall skin health.

Women's Health

Probiotics are of particular interest to women's health due to their potential to support vaginal health and prevent conditions like bacterial vaginosis and yeast infections. Lactobacillus strains are commonly found in the vaginal microbiome and can be taken as probiotic supplements to restore and maintain the balance of beneficial bacteria. Probiotics may also have a role in promoting overall women's health by maintaining gut health, which can have far-reaching effects on the body.

Allergies And Asthma

Emerging research suggests that early exposure to probiotics, both during pregnancy and infancy, may have a role in reducing the risk of allergies and asthma. Probiotics may help regulate the immune system's response to allergens, making it less likely to overreact and trigger allergic reactions or asthma symptoms.

While more studies are needed in this area, the potential for probiotics to play a preventive role in these conditions is an exciting prospect.

probiotics offer a wide range of potential benefits, impacting not only digestive health but also the immune system, mental well-being, skin health, women's health, and even the management of allergies and asthma.

As the field of probiotics continues to evolve, ongoing research will help us better understand their mechanisms and refine their applications for various health concerns, potentially opening up new avenues for improving human well-being.

CHAPTER THREE

Choosing The Right Probiotic Supplement

Selecting the right probiotic supplement can be a daunting task, given the multitude of products available in the market. Probiotics are live microorganisms that can provide various health benefits when consumed in adequate amounts.

They are often used to support digestive health, boost the immune system, and address a range of other health issues. However, not all probiotics are created equal, and several factors need to be considered to ensure you choose the most suitable supplement for your specific needs.

Factors To Consider

Strain Selection: Probiotics come in various strains, and each strain may have different health benefits. It's essential to identify the specific strain that targets your health concern.

For instance, Lactobacillus acidophilus may be beneficial for digestive issues, while Bifidobacterium bifidum is more suitable for immune support. Consulting a healthcare professional can help you determine the right strain for your condition.

CFUs (Colony-Forming Units): The number of live bacteria in a probiotic supplement is measured in CFUs. Higher CFU counts don't necessarily mean a better product, as the appropriate dosage depends on the intended use. Research the recommended CFU count for your condition, and choose a supplement that meets that requirement.

Viability: Probiotics are delicate microorganisms that can be killed by heat, humidity, and exposure to air and light. Ensuring the viability of the probiotics throughout their shelf life is crucial. Look for products that are specially formulated to protect probiotics from environmental factors, such as moisture-resistant packaging and enteric coatings to survive stomach acid.

Quality and Purity: A reputable manufacturer should produce the probiotic supplement under controlled conditions. Third-party testing for quality and purity is essential to guarantee that the product contains the specified strains and CFUs and is free from contaminants. Look for certifications like Good Manufacturing Practice (GMP) and the United States Pharmacopeia (USP) to ensure product quality.

Expiration Date: Always check the expiration date on the probiotic supplement. Using an expired product may not provide the expected health benefits since the probiotic bacteria may have died or diminished in potency.

Allergen Information: Some probiotic supplements may contain allergens like dairy, soy, or gluten. If you have food allergies or sensitivities, carefully read the ingredient list to ensure the supplement is safe for you.

Probiotic Delivery Systems

Probiotic supplements are available in various forms, and the choice of delivery system can impact their effectiveness. Common delivery systems include:

Capsules and Tablets: These are the most traditional forms of probiotic supplements and are easy to consume. They often have enteric coatings to protect probiotics from stomach acid, ensuring they reach the intestines alive.

Powders: Probiotic powders can be mixed with water, yogurt, or other liquids, providing flexibility in dosing. They are especially useful for children or individuals who have difficulty swallowing pills.

Chewables: Chewable tablets are designed to be more palatable and can be suitable for those who have trouble swallowing pills. However, they may contain added sugars or sweeteners, which can affect the product's overall health benefits.

Liquids: Probiotic liquids are typically easier to swallow, making them ideal for those who have difficulty with solid forms. However, they may have a shorter shelf life due to increased exposure to air and moisture.

• Fermented Foods: Natural sources of probiotics include yogurt, kefir, sauerkraut, kimchi, and other fermented foods. While these are a good dietary source of probiotics, it can be challenging to determine the exact probiotic content, making it less precise than supplements.

Choosing the right delivery system depends on personal preference, ease of use, and the specific needs of the individual. It's important to remember that the effectiveness of a probiotic supplement is not solely determined by its form but also by the viability and quality of the probiotic strains it contains.

Storage And Shelf Life

Proper storage of probiotic supplements is crucial to maintain their viability and efficacy. Here are some key considerations:

Temperature: Store probiotics in a cool, dry place away from direct sunlight and heat. High temperatures can kill probiotic bacteria. Some probiotic supplements require refrigeration to maintain their potency, so always follow the manufacturer's storage instructions.

Moisture: Moisture can activate probiotics prematurely or promote bacterial growth. Ensure the container is tightly sealed and moisture-resistant. Refrigerators can be excessively humid, so keep them in an airtight container within the fridge if required.

Exposure to Air and Light: Oxygen and light can also degrade probiotics over time. Choose supplements with opaque or dark-colored bottles to protect against light exposure, and make sure to reseal the container tightly after use.

Proper Sealing: Check the packaging for tamper-evident seals, which guarantee that the product hasn't been opened or compromised before purchase.

choosing the right probiotic supplement involves careful consideration of factors such as strain selection, CFU count, viability, quality, and delivery system. Additionally, proper storage and attention to shelf life are vital to ensure that you receive the maximum health benefits from your chosen probiotic supplement. Always consult with a healthcare professional to determine the most suitable product for your individual health needs.

Probiotics In Practice:

Probiotics have gained significant attention in recent years due to their potential health benefits.

These live microorganisms, typically bacteria or yeast, are known for their ability to confer various advantages to the human body when consumed in adequate amounts. Probiotics work by promoting a balanced and healthy gut microbiome, which plays a crucial role in supporting overall well-being.

When it comes to probiotics in practice, incorporating them into your daily routine can be a smart choice for maintaining and improving your health.

Probiotics can be found in various forms, including dietary supplements, fermented foods, and even prescription medications. One of the key aspects of using probiotics effectively is understanding which strains are best suited to your individual needs. Different strains of probiotics may offer distinct benefits, such as improved digestion, immune support, and relief from certain gastrointestinal issues. Consulting with a healthcare professional or a registered dietitian can help you make informed choices regarding probiotic strains and dosage.

CHAPTER FOUR

Integrating Probiotics Into Your Daily Routine:

Incorporating probiotics into your daily routine can be relatively straightforward, but it's essential to do so with some planning and understanding.

Probiotics can be found in various foods, such as yogurt, kefir, sauerkraut, and kimchi, making it easy to add them to your diet. Additionally, probiotic supplements are widely available and can offer a more convenient way to ensure a consistent intake of specific strains.

When selecting probiotic foods or supplements, it's essential to read labels and consider the strains included. Lactobacillus and Bifidobacterium are some of the most commonly used probiotic strains, but many others exist, each with its unique benefits. Moreover, the colony-forming units (CFUs) count on the packaging indicates the number of live microorganisms per serving.

Higher CFU counts may be suitable for specific health goals, but it's vital to seek guidance from a healthcare professional to determine the right dose for your specific needs.

The timing of probiotic consumption can also affect their effectiveness. For instance, taking probiotics with a meal may enhance their survival in the stomach's acidic environment and ensure they reach the intestines intact.

Over time, integrating probiotics into your daily routine can contribute to improved gut health, which, in turn, may positively impact various aspects of your well-being, from digestion to immune function.

Prebiotics And Synbiotics:

In the quest for a healthier gut, prebiotics and synbiotics play pivotal roles alongside probiotics. Prebiotics are non-digestible fibers found in various foods like garlic, onions, and certain fruits and vegetables.

They serve as nourishment for the beneficial bacteria in your gut, essentially acting as fuel for probiotics. By including prebiotic-rich foods in your diet, you can create an environment that promotes the growth and activity of probiotics.

On the other hand, synbiotics are a combination of probiotics and prebiotics. These products are specifically designed to deliver both live beneficial microorganisms and the fibers that support their growth.

The synergy between probiotics and prebiotics in synbiotics can enhance their effectiveness in promoting gut health.

Integrating prebiotics and synbiotics into your daily routine can be as simple as adding fiber-rich foods to your diet, such as whole grains, legumes, and fruits. This complements your probiotic consumption and supports the health of your gut microbiome, which is increasingly recognized as a critical factor in overall health.

Probiotics For Special Populations:

Probiotics are not a one-size-fits-all solution, and their benefits can vary depending on the individual and their specific health needs.

For special populations, such as infants, the elderly, or those with specific medical conditions, the use of probiotics may require careful consideration.

In infants, probiotics are sometimes recommended to promote a balanced gut microbiome, which can be particularly important for those born prematurely or delivered via C-section.

However, it's crucial to use probiotics in consultation with a pediatrician, as the choice of strains and dosage may differ based on the infant's health status.

For the elderly, probiotics can be beneficial in promoting digestive health, nutrient absorption, and potentially immune function.

Aging is often associated with changes in the gut microbiome, and probiotics may help mitigate these changes.

Still, individual health concerns and medications should be taken into account when considering probiotic supplementation in older adults.

In individuals with specific medical conditions, such as irritable bowel syndrome (IBS) or inflammatory bowel disease (IBD), probiotics may offer symptom relief and improved gut health.

However, the selection of probiotic strains and dosages should be tailored to the individual's condition and guided by a healthcare professional.

Integrating probiotics into your daily routine, understanding the roles of prebiotics and symbiotic and considering probiotics for special populations all require a thoughtful and informed approach.

 While probiotics offer promising health benefits, their effective use depends on factors such as strain selection, dosage, and individual health considerations. Consulting with a healthcare professional or registered dietitian can help you make the best choices for your specific needs, promoting a healthier gut and overall well-being.

Probiotics And Science

Probiotics have gained significant attention in recent years due to their potential health benefits. These microorganisms, primarily bacteria and some yeast strains, are often associated with maintaining a balanced and healthy gut microbiome.

The science behind probiotics revolves around understanding their role in supporting digestive health, immune function, and even their potential impact on various medical conditions.

As we delve into this topic, it's essential to explore the clinical research and studies that underpin the use of probiotic supplements, as well as consider their safety and side effects, all of which are subject to regulatory oversight.

CHAPTER FIVE

Clinical Research And Studies

Clinical research plays a pivotal role in establishing the scientific basis for probiotics. Numerous studies have focused on the impact of probiotics on different aspects of health, with the gut microbiome at the forefront. These studies often involve the administration of specific probiotic strains to evaluate their effects on gastrointestinal disorders, such as irritable bowel syndrome (IBS), inflammatory bowel disease (IBD), and antibiotic-associated diarrhea. Researchers have also investigated the potential benefits of probiotics for conditions beyond the gut, such as allergies, respiratory infections, and mental health.

Several clinical trials have highlighted the effectiveness of certain probiotic strains in alleviating symptoms associated with these conditions. For instance, Lactobacillus rhamnosus GG has shown promise in managing acute gastroenteritis in children, while Bifidobacterium infantis has demonstrated potential in mitigating symptoms of irritable bowel syndrome. However, it's important to note that the effectiveness of probiotics can vary depending on the specific strain, dosage, and the health condition being addressed. Moreover, research in the field of probiotics is ongoing, and new discoveries continue to shape our understanding of their potential benefits.

Safety And Side Effects

The safety profile of probiotics is a subject of concern, particularly in vulnerable populations, such as infants, the elderly, and individuals with compromised immune systems.

While probiotics are generally considered safe for healthy individuals, adverse effects, though rare, have been reported. These may include gastrointestinal symptoms like bloating, gas, and diarrhea. In more severe cases, probiotics can lead to infections, particularly in individuals with weakened immune defenses.

The risk of adverse effects varies depending on the strain of probiotic, the patient population, and the overall health of the individual. For example, individuals with short bowel syndrome or central venous catheters may be at higher risk for infections linked to probiotic use.

It is essential for healthcare providers to weigh the potential benefits against the risks when recommending probiotics for specific patients. Additionally, understanding the proper dosage and strain selection is crucial in minimizing the likelihood of side effects.

Regulatory Oversight

Probiotic supplements, as well as foods fortified with probiotics, are subject to regulatory oversight in many countries. These regulations are in place to ensure product safety and efficacy.

In the United States, the Food and Drug Administration (FDA) regulates probiotics as dietary supplements, which means they are not held to the same rigorous standards as pharmaceuticals. This lack of standardized regulation has led to some concerns about the consistency and quality of probiotic products.

In contrast, countries like Canada and some European nations have established specific guidelines and requirements for probiotics, which may include strain identification and product labeling. These regulatory measures are designed to enhance product transparency and safety.

Despite variations in regulations worldwide, the International Scientific Association for Probiotics and Prebiotics (ISAPP) has worked towards establishing global standards for probiotic research and product development. Their efforts aim to ensure that probiotics are well-researched, properly identified, and accurately labeled.

This not only helps consumers make informed choices but also fosters scientific credibility in the field.

probiotics represent a fascinating intersection of science, clinical research, safety considerations, and regulatory oversight. Their potential to impact various aspects of health has generated significant interest and continues to be an area of active investigation.

While probiotics hold promise in promoting well-being, it is essential to approach their use with caution, especially in vulnerable populations, and to rely on the best available scientific evidence to guide their consumption.

Furthermore, ongoing regulatory efforts aim to create a standardized framework for the production and marketing of probiotic products, enhancing their quality and safety for consumers.

Homemade Fermented Foods

Homemade fermented foods have gained significant popularity in recent years, largely due to the increasing awareness of the importance of probiotics for gut health and overall well-being.

Fermentation is a natural and age-old process that involves the transformation of food by beneficial microorganisms like bacteria, yeasts, and molds.

The result is a range of tasty and nutritious foods packed with live probiotic cultures. These homemade fermented foods are not only delicious but also offer numerous health benefits.

The key idea behind homemade fermented foods is to harness the power of beneficial microorganisms to preserve and enhance the nutritional value of the ingredients. Traditional fermented foods from various cultures worldwide include sauerkraut, kimchi, kombucha, kefir, yogurt, miso, and sourdough bread.

These foods undergo a controlled fermentation process, converting sugars and starches into lactic acid, alcohol, or other organic compounds, which contribute to their unique flavors and health-promoting properties.

Cultivating Your Own Probiotics

Cultivating your own probiotics at home is an exciting and cost-effective way to incorporate beneficial bacteria into your diet.

It allows you to have greater control over the fermentation process, ingredients, and flavors of the final product.

To get started, you need a starter culture containing live probiotics, which can be obtained from previous batches of fermented foods, a friend, or a trusted source. Common starters include sourdough starters, kefir grains, and yogurt cultures.

The fermentation process requires creating the right conditions for probiotic bacteria to thrive.

This typically involves controlling factors like temperature, time, and the composition of the ingredients.

The use of fermentation vessels like crocks, mason jars, and specialized containers can help maintain a controlled environment for these microorganisms. Additionally, it's essential to follow proper hygiene practices to ensure the growth of the intended beneficial bacteria while preventing the growth of harmful pathogens.

Fermented Food Recipes

Fermented food recipes are as diverse as the cultures from which they originate. There are numerous recipes available for creating homemade fermented foods that are not only rich in probiotics but also bursting with flavor. Let's explore a few examples:

Sauerkraut: To make this classic fermented cabbage dish, shred cabbage, mix it with salt, and then pack it into a clean jar. Allow it to ferment at room temperature for several days, and you'll have a tangy and crunchy sauerkraut.

Kombucha: Kombucha is a popular fermented tea beverage. It's made by fermenting sweet tea with a symbiotic culture of bacteria and yeast (SCOBY). The result is a fizzy and slightly sour drink with a unique flavor profile.

Yogurt: Homemade yogurt is made by introducing specific strains of bacteria, such as Lactobacillus bulgaricus and Streptococcus thermophilus, to warm milk. This simple process yields a creamy and probiotic-rich yogurt that can be flavored or enjoyed plain.

Kimchi: This Korean favorite involves fermenting Napa cabbage, radishes, and other vegetables with a spicy seasoning mixture. The outcome is a pungent, spicy, and sour side dish.

These are just a few examples, and the possibilities are nearly endless. Experimenting with ingredients and flavors can lead to unique creations that suit your taste preferences.

Safety And Quality Control

While the world of homemade fermented foods is exciting and rewarding, it's essential to emphasize safety and quality control to ensure that your creations are safe to consume. Here are some key points to consider:

Cleanliness: Maintaining a clean kitchen environment and using sanitized equipment is crucial to prevent the growth of harmful bacteria and ensure the intended probiotics flourish.

Proper Fermentation Conditions: Controlling factors like temperature and time is important to ensure a safe and delicious end product. Fermentation at too high or too low temperatures can lead to spoilage or undesirable flavors.

Ingredients: Use fresh and high-quality ingredients, and avoid any that may contain pesticides or preservatives that could hinder the fermentation process.

Observation: Keep an eye on your fermenting creations. If you notice any signs of mold, off-putting odors, or other abnormalities, it's essential to discard the batch to prevent potential health risks.

Storage: Properly store your fermented foods in the refrigerator or other appropriate storage conditions to extend their shelf life and maintain their probiotic content.

Homemade fermented foods can be a delicious and nutritious addition to your diet, providing valuable probiotics that can support your digestive health.

By understanding the principles of fermentation, cultivating your own probiotics, exploring a variety of recipes, and ensuring safety and quality control, you can embark on a journey of self-sufficiency in creating these flavorful and health-enhancing treats right in your own kitchen.

CHAPTER SIX

Probiotics And The Future

Probiotics, the live microorganisms that offer various health benefits when consumed, have garnered significant attention in recent years, and their role in shaping the future of healthcare and wellness is undeniable. As we delve into the emerging trends in probiotics, it becomes evident that the science and applications of these beneficial bacteria are continually evolving to address a wide array of health issues.

Emerging Trends

One of the most noteworthy emerging trends in the field of probiotics is their expanded application beyond traditional gut health. While probiotics have long been recognized for their role in maintaining digestive health, recent research has unveiled their potential in managing a broader spectrum of conditions. Studies are now exploring probiotics' impact on conditions such as mood disorders, allergies, and even skin health. This expansion of probiotics' scope points to a promising future in which they may become integral to holistic healthcare approaches.

Another trend gaining momentum is the identification and isolation of novel probiotic strains. Scientists are isolating specific strains with unique properties, which can be tailored to address specific health concerns. This trend dovetails with the growing popularity of personalized medicine, as it allows for the customization of probiotic treatments based on an individual's unique health profile.

The Role Of Genetics

Understanding the role of genetics in probiotic efficacy is a critical aspect of the evolving field. Genomic research has enabled scientists to investigate how an individual's genetic makeup can influence their response to probiotic interventions.

Genetic variations can impact the composition of the gut microbiome and how it interacts with probiotics, ultimately affecting their effectiveness. This knowledge is instrumental in developing targeted probiotic therapies that consider a person's genetic predisposition and microbiome composition.

Additionally, genetic insights are essential in predicting and managing adverse effects of probiotics. Some individuals may experience side effects or worsened symptoms when taking certain probiotics due to genetic factors. By tailoring probiotic recommendations to an individual's genetics, healthcare providers can minimize potential negative outcomes and enhance the overall safety and effectiveness of probiotic interventions.

Personalized Probiotics

The concept of personalized probiotics is at the forefront of probiotic research and application. As our understanding of the human microbiome and genetics advances, the potential for tailoring probiotics to an individual's unique health needs becomes increasingly viable. Personalized probiotics involve selecting specific probiotic strains, dosages, and treatment durations based on an individual's health history, genetics, and current health status. This approach aims to optimize the therapeutic benefits while minimizing potential risks.

Personalized probiotics have the potential to revolutionize healthcare by providing highly targeted and effective interventions for various health conditions. This approach may lead to more precise treatments for conditions such as irritable bowel syndrome, inflammatory bowel disease, and even mental health disorders, offering new hope for those who have not responded to conventional treatments.

Conclusion

The future of probiotics is characterized by remarkable growth and innovation. Emerging trends indicate that probiotics are poised to extend their applications well beyond traditional digestive health, offering solutions for an array of health issues. The integration of genetics into probiotic research and application is crucial for understanding how these beneficial bacteria interact with an individual's unique genetic makeup and microbiome composition. Personalized probiotics represent a transformative approach that has the potential to revolutionize healthcare by providing highly customized and effective interventions. As the field of probiotics continues to evolve, it holds great promise for improving human health and well-being in increasingly precise and individualized ways. Probiotics are on the cusp of transforming the landscape of healthcare and wellness, offering exciting prospects for the future.

www.ingramcontent.com/pod-product-compliance
Lightning Source LLC
Chambersburg PA
CBHW060805260726

48660CB00002B/783